Table of Contents

Sample 3-day meal plan

On the Volumetrics Diet, you should eat 3 meals per day, plus 2–3 snacks. Here's a 3-day sample menu:

Day 1

- Breakfast: oatmeal with fruit and a glass of skim milk
- Snack: carrots with hummus
- Lunch: grilled chicken with quinoa and asparagus
- Snack: sliced apples and light string cheese
- Dinner: baked cod with spiced vegetable couscous

Day 2

- Breakfast: nonfat yogurt with strawberries and blueberries
- Snack: a hard-boiled egg with tomato slices
- Lunch: turkey chili with kidney beans and vegetables
- Snack: a fruit salad with melon, kiwi, and strawberries
- Dinner: zucchini boats stuffed with ground beef, tomatoes, bell peppers, and marinara sauce

Day 3

- Breakfast: scrambled eggs with mushrooms, tomatoes, and onions, plus a slice of whole wheat toast
- Snack: a smoothie with skim milk, banana, and berries

- Lunch: chicken noodle soup with a side salad
- Snack: air-popped popcorn
- Dinner: whole grain pasta with turkey meatballs and sautéed vegetables

The meal plan above provides some simple meal and snack ideas for the Volumetrics Diet.

Will Volumetrics Diet help you lose weight?

You will very likely lose weight following the Volumetrics plan. In general, diets rich in low-energy-dense foods have been shown to promote fullness on fewer calories and deliver weight loss, according to the Centers for Disease Control and Prevention. Several systematic reviews and meta-analyses of observational studies have found lower-energy-dense diets to be associated with lower body weights.

There may even be hope for those who aren't big fans of veggies. For those who may not love the taste of vegetables, researchers investigated whether adding puréed vegetables to decrease the energy density of meals and increase daily vegetable intakes would help with weight loss. Over three weeks, 41 adults ate their breakfast, lunch and dinner at a lab. Some received the standard version of each meal; others got meals with 75% or 85% of the standard energy density by the addition of puréed veggies. Participants rated their hunger and fullness before and after meals. The meals with puréed veggies decreased daily calorie intake between 200 and 360 calories. Despite the decreased energy intake, ratings of hunger and fullness didn't significantly differ across the three groups. Entrées were rated as similar in palatability across conditions. The researchers concluded that adding pureed veggies can lead to substantial reductions in energy intake and increases in vegetable intake, reported in a 2011 issue of the American Journal of Clinical Nutrition.

Here's what several key studies had to say about Volumetrics and weight loss:

- A 2014 Drexel University study published in the journal Obesity looked at a variety of weight loss methods, including the Volumetrics approach of eating low-energy-dense foods. While all 132 participants in the study lost weight, the ones following a Volumetrics eating plan had "a superior outcome," having the greatest success in keeping the weight off even two years after the termination of the study.

- In a study published in the American Journal of Clinical Nutrition in 2007, researchers randomly assigned 97 obese women to either a low-fat diet or a low-energy-dense, low-fat diet that emphasized fruits and vegetables. After a year, both groups lost weight, but the fruits-and-vegetables dieters lost even more −14 pounds compared with 11 pounds. The researchers deemed low-energy-dense diets an effective way to drop pounds and keep them off.
- In another study, co-authored by Rolls, researchers investigated ways to maximize weight loss on a low-density diet. Two hundred overweight and

obese adults were placed on a low-density diet and divvied into four groups: one got a serving of soup a day, another got two servings of soup and a third got two daily snacks, like crackers or pretzels. (Soup, a high-water, low-density food, is a staple on the Volumetrics eating plan.) People in a fourth comparison group shaped their own low-density diet, without any special food instructions. After one year, those who supplemented their daily menu with one soup serving lost 13 2/5 pounds, compared with 15 9/10 for the two-soup group, 10 3/5 for the two-snack group and 17 9/10 for the comparison group, according to findings published in Obesity Research in 2005. Though the exact number of pounds lost varied, the study suggests that a diet high in low-density foods leads to substantial weight loss.

- In a study of 186 women, researchers found that those on higher-energy-density diets gained about 14 pounds over six years, while those on lower-energy-density diets gained 5 1/2 pounds, according to findings published in 2008 in the American Journal of Clinical Nutrition. The high-density group also saw their body mass index, a measure of body fat, increase more than the low-density group did. The findings suggest that decreasing energy density is a way to prevent weight gain and obesity in both the short and long term, the researchers concluded.

- Finally, in 2016, more research bolstered the link between low-density foods and weight loss. A systematic review of 13 studies, published in April in the journal Nutrients, found a significant association between low-energy-density foods and body weight reduction. In October, another study released online in the European Journal of Nutrition (and co-authored by Rolls) looked at food-consumption patterns in more than 9,500 adults. People with higher proportions of low- and very-low-energy-density foods in their diets had lower BMIs, smaller waist sizes and were less likely to be obese.

How easy is Volumetrics Diet to follow?

You won't go hungry on Volumetrics daily menus are designed to be filling, and include snacks and dessert. The focus is on making smart, sustainable tweaks to your eating habits that lower the overall caloric density of your diet. And since Volumetrics doesn't ban or severely limit entire food groups, your chances of sticking with it are higher.

Volumetrics offers convenience.

You're free to eat out, as long as you follow the diet's guidelines. Alcohol is OK in moderation. Volumetrics books make shaping your plan easier, but there's no way to avoid the grocery store and stove.

There are plenty of Volumetrics recipes to choose from.

There are Hundreds of recipes for appetizers, soups, sandwiches, pasta and vegetarian dishes (modified to cut energy density) . Choices include: roasted lamb chops, broccoli and tomato stuffed shells, and raspberry-apple crumble. Each has counts on calories, energy density and carbohydrate, fat, protein and fiber grams. Learn to lower the energy-density of traditional macaroni and cheese, for example, by using whole-wheat pasta, vegetables and low-fat cheese.

Eating out is allowed by the Volumetrics approach. Going out to eat is allowed by Volumetrics, you'll just have to determine which menu choices best conform. Starting with a low-calorie soup or salad makes you less likely to scarf your entire entree.

Volumetrics provides no timesavers.

The eating regimen offers no timesavers, unless you hire somebody to plan your meals, shop for them and prepare them. And you can't pay someone to exercise for you.

The eating plan does, however, provide some extras.which contain meal planning, grocery shopping and dining out guides; a crash course in nutrition basics; and advice for staying motivated.

Feeling full shouldn't be an issue.

Volumetrics was designed to promote satiety, the satisfied feeling that you've had enough. You shouldn't feel hungry on the diet, provided you adhere to its guidelines. Fruits, vegetables, soup and other low-density foods help control appetite, as do lean protein choices like poultry, seafood, tofu and beans.

There's no need to compromise on taste.

You don't have to give up your favorites with Volumetrics just make smart swaps. If you leave the butter off your bread, for example, you can have two slices instead of one for the same amount of calories. Or choose skim milk instead of whole and chug a larger glass for equal calories. And a morning stack of pancakes is still OK; just cut the oil and butter, switch to whole-wheat flour, use raspberry sauce instead of syrup and add fresh fruit on top. Other meal ideas range from a baked potato topped with veggies, salsa and cheese to chicken fajita pizza.

Does Volumetrics Diet have any health risks?

No indications of serious risks or side effects have surfaced. And there are no specific age restrictions: Volumetrics is safe for children and teens, too.

Is Volumetrics Diet a heart-healthy diet?

Yes, Volumetrics reflects the medical community's widely accepted definition of a heart healthy diet. An eating pattern heavy on fruits, veggies and whole grains but light on saturated fat and salt is considered the best way to keep cholesterol and blood pressure in check and heart disease at bay. In the 2005 Obesity Review study, the 200 participants following a low-density diet all showed significant drops in blood pressure (high blood pressure increases the risk of heart disease). Average blood pressure decreased from an already-normal 116/77 millimeters of mercury to 111/73 millimeters of mercury six months later, where it stayed for the duration of the yearlong study.

Can Volumetrics Diet prevent or control diabetes?

Being overweight is one of the biggest risk factors for Type 2 diabetes. If Volumetrics helps you lose weight and keep it off, you'll almost certainly tilt the odds in your favor. Most experts consider an eating pattern like what Volumetrics promotes to be the gold standard of diabetes prevention it emphasizes the right foods and discourages the wrong ones. And because there are no rigid meal plans or prepackaged meals, you can ensure that what you're eating doesn't go against your doctor's advice.

A 2017 observational study, published in the Journal of the Academy of Nutrition and Dietetics, followed more than 143,000 women for roughly 12 years. Risk of developing Type 2 diabetes was 24% greater for women who ate diets higher in energy density compared with women who followed a lower-energy-dense diet.

A study published in 2007 in Diabetes Care found that adults following an eating plan resembling Volumetrics had significantly lower fasting insulin levels than those whose diets emphasized high-energy-dense food. Low-density diets, the authors wrote, help prevent insulin resistance a frequent precursor to Type 2 diabetes in which the body doesn't respond as it should to the hormone.

Does Volumetrics Diet allow for restrictions and preferences?

Anyone can follow Volumetrics choose your preference for more information.

Supplement recommended? No.

Vegetarian or Vegan: The bulk of what you'll be eating fruits, vegetables and whole grains are staples of both vegetarian and vegan diets.

Gluten-Free: People who can't tolerate gluten, a protein found in wheat, barley and rye, can easily adapt Volumetrics to fit their needs.

Low-Salt: It's up to you to make sure your choices are low-sodium, but such a heavy emphasis on fruits and veggies (stick with fresh or sodium-free frozen) should make your job easier. It'll also help that you're eating meat and dairy often high-sodium culprits in moderation.

Kosher: Yes, you have the freedom to use only kosher ingredients.

Halal: Yes, but it's up to you to ensure your food conforms.

Is Volumetrics Diet nutritious?

Volumetrics is based on low-energy-density foods. Its menu items are large in volume but low in calories. That's thanks to a whole lot of fruits, vegetables, whole grains, nonfat dairy and lean meat. Volumetrics fully or almost meets recommendations for the majority of necessary nutrients, making it a safe and healthy way of eating.

The Volumetrics diet and health

While more analysis is needed on the role of energy density in weight management and the prevention of overweight and obesity, there is research supporting the use of a low-energy-dense diet to improve appetite control and help achieve weight-loss goals. By emphasizing whole foods and personalization of the diet rather than cutting out entire food groups or placing strict rules on food consumption, the Volumetrics diet is likely to be a more sustainable eating pattern than popular, uick-fix fad diets.

Some research has also been done on the connection between energy density and specific health outcomes:

- Cardiovascular disease: Some research suggeststhe potential for a low-energy-dense diet to benefit factors affecting cardiovascular disease, but sufficient evidence is lacking to fully support this.
- Type 2 diabetes: In a large observational study, women who ate diets higher in energy density had a higher risk of developing type 2 diabetes as compared with women who followed a lower-energy-dense diet.
- Breast cancer: One large observational study determined that women who had the highest-energy-dense diet had a higher risk for postmenopausal breast cancer compared with women who followed the lowest energy-dense diet.

- Weight loss: Several systematic reviews and meta-analyses of observational studies have found lower-energy-dense diets to be associated with lower body weights. Evidence from randomized controlled trials have also shown lower-energy-dense diets to be helpful for weight management and weight loss maintenance.

WEIGHT LOSS WONDER SOUP

INGREDIENTS

- 1/2 tsp olive oil, optional
- 4 large onions, finely chopped (6-8 coups)
- 2 green peppers, diced (2-3 cups)
- 3 large tomatoes, roughly chopped (3-4 cups)
- 1 bunch celery, diced (3-4 cups)
- 1 small cabbage, chopped (10-12 cups)3 cup water, or up to 5 cups for a more watery soup

Preparation

- Start off by cutting up all the vegetables and separating them into three large bowls: onion and green pepper in the first bowl, tomatoes and celery in the second bowl, and cabbage in the last bowl.
- In a large skillet, heat olive oil over medium-high heat. Add onions and green peppers to pan, tossing to coat. Sautee veggies until water has cooked out and onions begin to brown. The length of time this takes will depend on your cooking unit and the size of your pan, but for me, it took about 35 minutes. Turn the veggies every 3 to 5 minutes while cooking to prevent sticking and to check the color. Once cooked, remove pan from heat.

- In a 12 quart stockpot, add the cabbage and water. Next, add the tomatoes and celery. Finish by adding the cooked onions and green peppers on top. Ingredients will likely be to be brim of the pot - this is okay. Do not stir soup yet.

- Heat the soup over medium-high until water begins to boil. By this point, the veggies should have cooked down some, giving you room to stir. Once veggies are mixed, reduce heat so soup is simmering and cook for 50-60 minutes, stirring occasionally.

- If desired, serve soup immediately. Store excess soup in a sealed container in the refrigerator for up to 5 days.

Brownie Pancakes with Berry Cream Sauce

Ingredients

PANCAKES

- 1/2 cup white whole-wheat flour
- 2 tablespoons cornstarch
- 2 tablespoons sugar
- 1-1/2 teaspoons baking powder
- 1/4 teaspoon table salt
- 1-1/4 cups 1% fat cottage cheese
- 3 large eggs
- 1 tablespoon melted butter or oil

SAUCE

- 3 cups frozen or fresh mixed berries strawberries or blueberries

- 1 tablespoon cornstarch
- 1 tablespoon sugar

Preparation

- Stir together the flour, cornstarch, sugar, baking powder and salt in a large bowl. Whisk together the cottage cheese, eggs and butter in a small bowl. Add to the flour mixture and stir to combine. It is okay for the batter to have a few small lumps.
- Heat a nonstick griddle or large skillet on the stove over medium-low heat. Place 2 tablespoons of batter on the griddle for each pancake, leaving

space for the pancakes to spread without touching each other. Flip the pancakes with a spatula when the bubbles on the top begin to pop and the bottom is dry. Cook for 1 or 2 minutes more, until the bottom is lightly browned.

- Meanwhile, toss the berries with the cornstarch and sugar in a medium microwaveable bowl. Microwave at 1-minute intervals, gently stirring between intervals, until the berries are soft and the liquid is bubbling and thickened, about 5 minutes.

High Volume Taco Meal Prep Bowls

Ingredients

Veggie Stir Fry

- 12 oz bag Frozen Cauliflower Rice
- 15 oz can Black Beans, drained and rinsed
- 15 oz can Whole Kernel Corn, drained and rinsed
- 2 medium Bell Peppers, I used a red and green
- 1-2 Jalapeño Peppers, optional
- 1/2-1 Tbsp Chili Powder, (to spice preference)

* 1 Tbsp Olive Oil, optional

Beef Taco Mixture

- 1 lb Ground Beef, I used 96/4 from HEB
- 1 medium (200g) Yellow Onion, diced
- 5 cloves (25g) Peeled Garlic, minced
- 2 tsp Paprika
- 1/2 tsp Kosher Salt
- 1/2 tsp Black Pepper
- 1/2 tsp Cumin
- 1/4-1 tsp Crushed or Ground Chipotle Pepper, or chili powder (to spice preference)
- 1/2 C (120g) Enchilada Sauce , or salsa
- 4 oz can Diced Green Chiles

Preparation

- Microwave the cauliflower rice for 4-5 minutes while you prep the bell pepper, jalapeño, onion, garlic, black beans, and corn.

- When all your vegetables are prepped, heat the olive oil in a large skillet over medium-high heat. Add the cauliflower rice, beans, corn, and peppers to the skillet. Briefly stir and then leave untouched for about 4-5 minutes to develop a bit of char on the bottom. Add the chili powder after 5 minutes and stir everything together. Continue cooking for another 5 minutes or so.

- Add the beef, onion, and garlic to a separate large skillet over medium-high heat and break the beef apart. Cook until no pink remains before reducing the heat to medium-low, adding the dry spices, enchilada sauce, and diced chiles. Simmer for about 5 minutes to let all the flavors get acquainted.

- To make the 4 meal prep bowls, add 1 cup or 200 grams of each mixture to a bowl or container. Squeeze a bit of fresh lime juice, garnish with cilantro, and add any other toppings you'd like when serving.

Instant Pot Weight Loss Soup

Ingredients

- 1 tablespoon extra-virgin olive oil
- 2 medium onions (chopped)
- 4 medium carrots (chopped)
- 4 stalks celery (chopped)
- 4 cloves garlic (minced)
- 4 cups chopped cabbage (half head)
- 1 green bell pepper (chopped)

- 1 zucchini (chopped)
- 1 14- ounce can diced tomatoes
- 8 cups bone broth (or low-sodium vegetable broth)
- 1 bay leaf
- 1 teaspoon oregano
- 1 teaspoon basil
- ½ teaspoon red pepper flakes
- 1 teaspoon salt (optional)
- 1/2 teaspoon black pepper

Preparation

- Set Instant Pot to the saute setting. Add the olive oil and allow to heat for 1 minute. Add the onion, carrots and celery and cook, stirring occasionally, until softened, 5 -7 minutes. Stir in the garlic and cook for 1 minute longer.

- Add the cabbage, green pepper, zucchini, tomatoes, broth, bay leaf, spices and salt and pepper. Stir to combine.

- Put the lid on the Instant Pot, close the steam vent and set to HIGH pressure using the manual setting. Decrease the time to 4 minutes. It will take about 15 minutes for the pressure to build, then the timer will start.

- Once the time is expired, wait for 5 minutes, then carefully use the quick release valve to release the steam. Season to taste with salt and pepper. Serve.

Susan's Dirty Little Secret Soup

Ingredients

- 5-6 cups vegetable broth I use Imagine No-Chicken
- 1 16- ounce can diced tomatoes
- 2 16- ounce cans beans rinsed and drained (I usually use 1 Great Northern and 1 Kidney Bean)
- 2 1- pound bags of frozen vegetables (my favorites are California Blend [cauliflower, broccoli, and carrots] and Italian Blend [zucchini, Italian green beans, broccoli, red pepper])
- 4 cloves minced garlic
- 1 teaspoon basil
- 1/2 teaspoons oregano
- 1/2 teaspoon thyme

- a shake or two of hot pepper sauce (Tabasco)
- black pepper and salt to taste
- 1/2 cup small pasta OR 2 cups diced potatoes OR 1 cup frozen corn or other starchy vegetable OR 1/2 cup of quick-cooking grain (buckwheat, pearled barley, millet, or quinoa or cooked rice OPTIONAL

Preparation

- Put 5 cups of vegetable broth and all remaining ingredients into a large pot. Bring to a boil, reduce heat, and simmer until vegetables are done, about 20-30 minutes. If the soup seems too thick, add more broth.

Taste and adjust seasonings before serving.

- This can also be made with 2 pounds of whatever fresh vegetables you have in the house.

Chicken Salad with Lemon-Ginger Dressing

INGREDIENTS

For the lemon-ginger dressing:

- ½ t lemon zest
- ½ c lemon juice, fresh squeezed
- 1 t grated ginger, fresh
- 2 T avocado oil
- salt and pepper, to taste

For the chicken salads:

- 8 c mixed salad greens
- 6 ounces cabbage, shredded
- 1 medium cucumber, chopped (mine was 13.6 ounces)
- 1 medium red pepper, chopped
- 1 c mandarin orange segments, drained
- 12 ounces grilled chicken, chopped (can substitute chopped rotisserie chicken breast)
- 4 scallions, sliced
- 2 ounces chopped cashews (approximately ½ cup)

Preparation

To make the lemon-ginger dressing:

- Place the zest, juice, ginger, oil, salt, and pepper in a one-cup canning jar. Put the lid on the jar and shake to combine the ingredients.
- Distribute the dressing evening between four dressing cups.
- To make the chicken salads:
- Distribute the mixed greens and cabbage evenly between four salad containers.
- Top the greens with the cucumber, pepper, oranges, and chicken. Try to distribute these ingredients evenly between the four containers.
- Garnish your salads with the scallions and cashews.

- You're all ready for lunch for the next four days!

Creamy Tomato Soup

Ingredients

- 2 tablespoons extra virgin olive oil, divided
- 1 large onion, chopped
- 4 garlic cloves, chopped
- 1 tablespoon tomato paste
- 1 (26.46-ounce) box of chopped or crushed Italian tomatoes
- 1/2 teaspoon coarse black pepper
- 2 1/2 cups vegetables broth
- 1 1/2 ounces Parmesan cheese

- 2 ounces bread (no seeds or nuts), torn into about 4 pieces
- 5 fresh basil leaves

Preparation

- Heat 1 tablespoon of olive oil in a large saucepan over medium heat. Add the onion and sauté about 5 minutes.
- Add the garlic and tomato paste. Stir.
- Add the tomatoes, black pepper and vegetable broth. Raise heat to high, and bring to a boil.
- Reduce the heat to low. Add the Parmesan cheese and bread. Cover and simmer for about 20 minutes.
- Remove from the heat. Add the basil leaves and 1 tablespoon olive oil.

Using an immersion blender (or a stand blender, with extra caution), puree the soup until smooth.

Cabbage Soup Diet Recipe

Ingredients

- 2 tbsp olive oil
- 1 yellow or white onion chopped
- 2 bell peppers chopped (any color)
- 4 celery stalks chopped
- 6 garlic cloves minced
- 2 large tomatoes chopped
- 1 cup broccoli slaw optional
- 1 green cabbage head chopped

- 9 cups low-sodium broth chicken or vegetable broth
- 1 tbsp tomato paste
- 1 tsp ground black pepper
- 1 tbsp ground turmeric
- 2 cups baby spinach
- 1 lemon juiced
- salt to taste

Preparation

- Instant Pot Cabbage Soup: To make the detox cabbage soup in the pressure cooker, press the saute function. Heat oil and cook onion, bell pepper, and celery for about 5 minutes, or until softened. Stir every now and then. Add garlic and cook for 1 minute. Add tomato, broccoli slaw, cabbage, broth, tomato paste, pepper, and turmeric. Stir and secure lid. Set on high for 15 minutes, or press the soup function and set for 15 minutes. Allow natural release, about 20 minutes. Remove lid and stir in spinach and lemon juice. Stir in salt but do not go overboard.

- Slow Cooker Cabbage Soup: Heat a large nonstick skillet over medium heat, add oil and cook onion, bell pepper, and celery for about 5 minutes, or until softened. Stir every now and then. Add garlic and cook for 1 minute. Transfer to the slow cooker. Stir in all the other ingredients for the cabbage soup diet recipe, except spinach, lemon juice, and salt. Secure lid and cook for 2-4 hours on high, or 8-10 hours on low. Remove lid and stir in spinach and lemon juice. Stir in salt but go easy.

- Cabbage Soup on the Stovetop: Heat a large nonstick pot or dutch oven over medium heat, add oil and cook onion, bell pepper, and celery for about 5 minutes, or until softened. Stir every now and then. Add garlic and cook for 1 minute. Stir in all the other ingredients, except spinach, lemon juice, and salt. Increase heat to medium-high and bring to a boil. Reduce heat to medium-low, stir, cover, and let simmer for 30 minutes, or until veggies are tender. Remove lid and stir in spinach and lemon juice. Stir in just enough salt to taste.

Healthy Bolognese Sauce

Ingredients

- 1 tablespoon olive oil
- 1 lb turkey
- 1.5 cup carrots minced finely
- 2 tablespoons garlic minced finely
- 1 cup onion minced finely
- 1 cup celery minced finely
- 56 oz cans crushed tomatoes (2 28 oz cans)
- 1/2 teaspoon salt
- 1 teaspoon pepper
- ¼ teaspoon red pepper flakes
- ¼ cup fresh basil chopped finely
- ¼ cup fresh parsley chopped finely

Preparation

Crockpot Instructions:

- In a pan, heat 1 tablespoon olive oil. Brown ground turkey for 5-7 minutes. When fully cooked, remove from pan and set aside, reserving the juices/grease
- Add carrots, garlic, onion and celery. Saute until onions are translucent, about 5 minutes.
- Add cooked ground turkey + veggies, along with tomatoes, spices + herbs into crockpot base
- Stir to combine. Cook on low for 8-10 hours or high for 4-6 hours.
- Serve over pasta, zucchini noodles, rice, or whatever you like best!

Rustic Sausage Vegetable Soup

Ingredients

- 1 link Smoked sausage - fully cooked (such as Aidell's). Choose chicken, pork, or kielbasa as you choose. Our stats are for 1 link of chicken apple sausage
- 3 tablespoons Extra Virgin Olive Oil
- 3 cloves Garlic
- 1/4 medium Onion - chopped
- 1 medium Potato - peeled and diced into small cubes
- 1 cup Peas - fresh or from frozen (see note)
- 1 cup Corn - fresh or from frozen

- 2 cups California Vegetable Blend - Cauliflower, Broccoli and Carrots - fresh or from frozen
- 2 cups Artichoke Hearts - frozen (not canned with oil or other ingredients)
- 2 cups Cabbage - rough chopped
- 1 cup Celery - rough chopped, including leaves
- 1 medium Tomato - rough chopped, seeds discarded
- 1 tablespoon Ranch Buttermilk Dressing powder - optional (see note)
- 1 tablespoon Au Jus Powder - optional (see note)
- 1 can Small White Beans - drained (such as Navy or Cannellini)
- 32 ounces Chicken Broth - low sodium
- 2 cups Water

Preparation

- In the Instant Pot 8 quart pot, select "saute" and add the olive oil.
- While the pot and oil are warming, chop up 1 medium link of low-fat smoked sausage into bite size and smaller pieces. This sausage is included for a bit of flavor as opposed to a major protein source.
- In the oil, saute the sausage pieces, the diced onion, and the garlic cloves, until soft, translucent and fragrant.
- Add in the chicken broth and water, and leave the pot on "saute mode" so that it begin to warm the broth and everything we now add (the majority of which was frozen).
- Chop the potato, celery and leaves, and tomato into small bite size pieces,

and add to the pot, stirring as you go, while it is still.

- Pour in the quantities given of the frozen vegetable blend, peas, corn, and frozen artichoke hearts. Add or subtract frozen vegetables of your choice as you go.
- Drain and rinse the canned beans, and add to the pot, stirring as you go.
- Add the chopped cabbage, stirring as you go.
- Now we begin to season. We have a container of Au Jus (dry) powder mixed with dried Buttermilk Ranch powder, and this is our "House Mississippi Blend" we use on chicken and roasts, so we added about 2 tablespoons of this (or you could use 1 teaspoon of each if you don't have it combined as we do).

- Now taste and add your favorite combo savory seasoning blend. We added 1-2 tablespoons of our favorite Spice Blend Of All Time (which we use on EVERYTHING savory it seems) Penzey's Ozark Seasoning. You can choose what YOU like perhaps it's chili seasoning, or curry, or even steak seasoning, so long as it isn't too high in sodium. The Ozark blend includes salt, Tellicherry black pepper, garlic, thyme, sage, paprika, mustard, ancho, celery, cayenne, dill weed, dill seed, caraway, allspice, ginger, cardamom, bay leaf, mace, cassia, savory, and cloves.

- Stir and taste your broth. It should be flavorful, but not overpowering, because you can always adjust when the soup is done.

- Cancel the "saute" mode and select "soup" mode. Set the timer for 30 minutes. Seal the pot with the lid.
- Release manually, remove the lid, and unplug the pot. You don't want the vegetables to get mushy during slow release. Stir and taste, and season as you like, with more spices if necessary.
- Serve and enjoy, and feel full and sated!

THAI CHICKEN ZUCCHINI NOODLES

INGREDIENTS

- 1 chicken breast
- salt & pepper
- 1 tablespoon coconut oil
- 1 large zucchini, peeled/spiralized (I used a julienne peeler)
- 1/4 cup cilantro, chopped
- 2 tablespoons cashews, chopped
- 1 carrot, chopped
- 1 tablespoon peanut butter
- 1/2 lime, juiced
- 1/2 tablespoon honey
- 2 tablespoons coconut cream from a can
- 1/2 tablespoon fish sauce
- 1 teaspoon ginger, minced

- 1 clove garlic, minced
- 1/2 tablespoon jalapeno, minced

Preparation

- Heat a skillet over medium high heat and melt coconut oil.
- Season chicken breast with salt & pepper and once hot, add to skillet.
- Cook for about 3-4 minutes per side until cooked through.
- Remove from skillet and shred, set aside.
- In a small bowl combine, peanut butter, lime juice, honey, coconut cream, fish sauce, ginger, garlic & jalapeno. Whisk together and set aside.

- Combine shredded chicken in a large bowl with peeled/spiralized zucchini, cilantro, cashews and carrots.
- Pour the sauce in the bowl and toss to combine.

Easy Banana Bread Recipe (Classic Banana Bread)

Ingredients

- 8 Tablespoons Unsalted Butter (softened)
- 2 Eggs (large)
- 3 Bananas (ripe & large sized)

- 2 Cups Flour (all purpose flour)
- 1 Cup White Granulated Sugar
- 1 Teaspoon Vanilla Extract
- 1 Teaspoon Baking Soda
- 1 Teaspoon Baking Powder (aluminum free)
- 1/2 Teaspoon Salt

Preparation

- Preheat oven to 325 degrees F.
- Mash bananas with a fork.
- Soften butter in a microwave.
- Stir eggs, bananas and butter together.
- Mix in remaining ingredients. Stir until the batter is fully mixed.

Optional – If you want to enhance this easy "basic" banana bread, you can stir in 1 cup of your family's favorite dessert ingredient (i.e. chocolate chips or chopped walnuts) after you have mixed the batter.

- Pour the finished batter into a nonstick bread pan. Smooth out the top of the batter within the bread pan.
- Bake in the oven for 65-70 minutes or until golden brown.
- Take out of oven and let the banana bread cool down in the bread pan for 10 minutes. Do not remove the banana bread from the bread pan during this 10 minute cool down period. Use oven mitts as the bread pan will be very hot coming out of the oven.

- After 10 minutes, remove the banana bread from the bread pan. Place the banana bread on a cooling rack in order to completely cool. This cool down may take 1-2 hours. Gently slide a silicon spatula between the banana bread and the bread pan walls if the banana bread is stuck in the pan.

www.ingramcontent.com/pod-product-compliance
Lightning Source LLC
Chambersburg PA
CBHW060809260726
48660CB00002B/849